getting into

Physiotherapy
Courses

trotman

getting into

Physiotherapy
Courses

James Burnett

£12.99

Getting into Physiotherapy Courses
Fourth edition

This fourth edition published in 2008 by Trotman Publishing, a division of Crimson Publishing Ltd.,
Westminster House, Kew Road, Richmond, Surrey TW9 2ND

© Trotman Publishing 2008

First Edition Published

Editorial and Publishing Team
Author James Burnett
Advertising Sarah Talbot, Advertising Sales Director

British Library Cataloguing in Publication Data
A catalogue record for this book is available from the British Library

ISBN 978 184455 150 7

Typeset by NewGen Imaging

Printed and bound by The Cromwell Press, Trowbridge, Wiltshire

Contents

For the latest news on physiotherapy and physiotherapy
courses, go to www.mpw.co.uk/getintomed

About the author

James Burnett is Director of Studies and a careers advisor at Mander Portman Woodward's London college, and he has sat on a number of university interview panels. He is the author of several books in the MPW "Getting into..." series, including "Getting into Medical School, "Getting into Dental School", and "Getting into Art and Design Courses". He has written a number of study guides, including "Surviving Year 12" published by Trotman; and has had articles published in careers publications and national newspapers. He is a past chairman of the Conference for Independent Further Education (CIFE).

Acknowledgements

I would like to thank Alice Holmes for her help in getting this project started, and Fiona Pyrgos at Bryanston School who arranged for us to talk to students who are now studying physiotherapy at university. I would also like to thank Katherine Cran, Tania Dawson and the other students who shared their experiences with us. Thank you also to Maya Waterstone for her help in compiling the data on entrance requirements, the university admissions staff who answered our questions, everyone at Trotman and Company for enabling us to write this book and, most importantly, the Chartered Society of Physiotherapy for the enormous amount of information they provided.

The information in this book has come from a variety of sources and is, we believe, correct at the time of going to press. However, the views expressed are our own and any errors are down to us.

James Burnett
December 2007

Introduction

Most people associate physiotherapy with sport. Footballers are reported to be 'seeing the physio' after an injury, and the sight of a tracksuited figure running onto the sports field carrying an aerosol spray and the 'magic' sponge when a player is lying on the ground is a common one. For others, physiotherapy is something that takes place after an accident when the victim needs to learn to walk properly. However, whilst physiotherapy encompasses both of these, there are many other facets to the profession.

■ What is physiotherapy?

The human body is a complex machine that can go wrong for any number of reasons. Physiotherapy is a science-based medical subject that looks in detail at how the body moves, how muscles, bones, joints and ligaments work and how they react to pain and trauma. Physiotherapists diagnose numerous ailments that affect the muscles and nerves, and then proceed to treat the patient, ensuring independence, movement and a return to maximum performance. It is the physiotherapist's job not only to look at the problem and treat it but also to look for any predisposing factors that may have contributed to the patient's ailment and to advise on how to minimise the risk of the same thing happening again. Qualified physiotherapists work independently and as part of multidisciplinary teams ensuring that patients' health and mobility are improved.

■ What do physiotherapists do?

Physiotherapists have numerous challenging roles within the health sector. They provide services such as rehabilitation and exercise before and after surgery. Within the wider community they provide services to adults with learning difficulties. They also have a role in the workplace where they can help to reduce injuries such as Repetitive Strain Injury (RSI).

Chartered physiotherapists work with a wide range of people in many different environments either individually or as part of a large healthcare team. Physiotherapists deal with many different situations, which include:

- Teaching people the 'correct' ways to move and lift, in order to prevent or to slow the onset of problems such as back pain and RSI – see *Useful Information*. This may include helping athletes to avoid injury by discussing techniques and training programmes. Poor warm-up routines, too much training, poor equipment and incorrect technique are common causes of injuries, all of which might be avoided. Using the idea that prevention is better than cure physiotherapists are able to show people that very small changes will be hugely beneficial, for example good footwear or the use of a wrist support when using a computer.

■ Helping women before and after pregnancy by advising them about posture and exercise.

■ Helping children to deal with mental and physical disabilities.

■ Developing the potential of people with learning difficulties through exercise, sport and recreation; this could also include the use of specialist equipment.

■ Helping people deal with stress and anxiety.

■ Helping stroke victims recover movement in paralysed limbs.

■ Helping orthopaedic patients after spinal operations or joint replacements and treating those debilitated following an accident. Using a variety of techniques to strengthen muscles and improve the mobility of individual joints, activities such as walking can be made much easier for people recovering from hip replacements or those with arthritis or osteoporosis. These methods can also reduce the pain and stiffness resulting from these conditions.

■ Working with AIDS patients.

■ Caring for the elderly who suffer from Parkinson's disease.

■ Improving the confidence and self-esteem of those with mental illness through exercise and recreation, whilst also helping with relaxation and body awareness techniques.

■ Working with the terminally ill or those in intensive care (inpatients and outpatients) to maintain movement and prevent respiratory problems.

■ Helping sportspeople recover from injury.

■ Working in large businesses and companies to ensure that employees do not suffer from physical problems associated with their jobs.

Physiotherapists use a range of techniques including:

■ Manipulation
■ Massage
■ Exercise
■ Hydrotherapy
■ Vibration
■ Ultrasound
■ Infrared and ultraviolet radiation.

'Physiotherapy appealed to me because it was a practical job, rather than being academically based. I had always been interested in science and biology in particular, and come from a medical

background. I had seen both my parents treat patients in different ways and get great satisfaction from it, and I felt it was something I wanted to do.'

Katherine, University of Hertfordshire

Physiotherapy is not, however, a profession that only involves physical therapy. Physiotherapists work with people – in most cases people who are disabled, or who have been ill or injured. Physiotherapists need to be able to communicate on a personal level with people of all ages; to be reassuring and comforting; to explain the treatments they are using; and to help patients to overcome fear and pain. Physiotherapists need to be able to assess the needs of their patients and to be aware of the effects of external circumstances such as social or cultural factors.

■ Working as a physiotherapist

Physiotherapists work in a range of health and care environments that include hospitals, the local community, private practice, industry and sports settings. The majority are employed by the NHS. Physiotherapy comprises the largest group within the allied healthcare professions with over 30,000 state-registered physiotherapists in the UK. To qualify as a registered physiotherapist you need to gain an approved degree (see page 51) that has been validated by the Chartered Society of Physiotherapy (CSP) and the Council for Professions Supplementary to Medicine (CPSM). If you complete the degree you are then eligible for state registration (SRP) and Membership of the Chartered Society of Physiotherapy (MCSP). Career prospects for physiotherapists are excellent, with most graduates finding employment as soon as they complete their university courses.

■ How to use this book

The competition for places on approved degree courses is intense – there are very few university courses that have more applicants per place than physiotherapy. There are more applicants per place for physiotherapy than for medicine, for veterinary science or for courses at Oxford or Cambridge. Typically a university might receive over 1000 applications for 40 places. Even if each applicant makes five choices – and not all do – this still works out at around five students chasing every place. As you will see on page 5, it is often far more than this. With such intense competition for places you need to think carefully about all stages of your application, from the preparation that you do before you apply through to the interview and the steps to take to maximise your chances of gaining a place should something go wrong at the examination stage.

This book is divided into four sections:

- Getting an interview
- Getting an offer
- Results day
- Useful information.

The first section deals with the preparation that you need to undertake in order to make your application as strong as possible. It includes advice on work experience, how to choose a university, and the UCAS application itself. The section on interviews provides tips on what to expect and on how to ensure that you come across as a potential physiotherapist. It also contains a checklist for you to tick off the important steps in making your application. The third section describes the steps that you need to take if you are holding an offer, or if you do not have an offer but want to gain a place through Clearing. The final section provides background information on physiotherapy and on physiotherapy issues.

Entry requirements are quoted in terms of A level grades or UCAS points (the UCAS tariff) in this book. Information for students with Scottish Highers, the International Baccalaureate (IB), the BTEC National Diploma or the Irish Leaving Certificate is on page 40. The universities will be happy to provide you with further information on other qualifications.

On pages 38–40 there is advice and information for 'non-standard' applicants – mature students, graduates and retake students.

As with other books in this series, including *Getting into Medical School* and *Getting into Dental School*, this book is designed to be a route map for potential physiotherapists rather than a guide to physiotherapy as a profession. The Chartered Society of Physiotherapy, or physiotherapists whom you meet during work experience, should be the starting points for more detailed information on what being a physiotherapist entails. You should also consult Trotman's career guide *Getting into Physiotherapy*.

For the latest news on physiotherapy and physiotherapy courses, go to www.mpw.co.uk/getintomed

---

01 Getting an interview

In order to gain a place at university you have to submit a UCAS application. Before you do this, however, you need to be sure that you have investigated physiotherapy as thoroughly as you can. You need to do this for two reasons:

- You must be sure that physiotherapy is the right career for you
- You must demonstrate to the university admissions tutors that you are aware of the demands of the profession.

With so many applicants for every university place the selectors need to be sure that they do not 'waste' a place on someone who will then drop out of the course or the profession. For this reason the application has to be very convincing. Most people's exposure to physiotherapy is limited, and so you need to investigate the profession in depth.

When your UCAS application is received by the university it will not be on its own, but in a batch of, possibly, several hundred. The selectors will have to consider it, along with the others, in between the demands of their 'real' jobs. If your application is uninteresting, lacking evidence of real commitment to physiotherapy, or badly worded, it will be put on the reject pile. Nottingham University, for example, receives more than 1600 applications for its 60 places. From these, about 300 people are interviewed. A useful step-by-step guide to the selection process used by Nottingham can be found at www.nottingham.ac.uk/chs/courses/physiotherapy-bsc.php.

You can only be called for interview on the basis of your UCAS application. The selectors will not know about the things that you have forgotten to say and they can only get an impression of you from what is in the application. We have come across too many good students who never got an interview simply because they did not think about the UCAS application: they relied on the hope that the selectors would somehow see through the words and get an instinctive feeling about them.

The following sections will tell you more about what the selectors are looking for, and how you can avoid common mistakes. Before looking at how the selectors go about deciding whom to call to interview, however, there are a number of important things that you need to think about.

'When we interview students, we want to find out two things – whether they are really committed to the profession, and whether they have the right personality to succeed. For the first of these, it is work experience, work experience, work experience that

matters. For the second, I look for the ability to respond to my questions calmly and with structure. I also look at whether they have contributed to the life of their school, college or community.'

Admissions tutor

■ Work experience

According to Nottingham University's physiotherapy website, 'your experience should give you a feel for the breadth, depth and requirements of the profession and for the personal qualities and characteristics that are necessary in a physiotherapist. It is important to note that without work experience it is likely that your application will be rejected automatically at the initial stages.'

Work experience is vital if you are to be considered. Without evidence that you have worked with people in the community, preferably within the NHS, you will not be offered a place. Although not all universities are as explicit as Nottingham most will emphasise the need for work experience. For example, Brunel University's website says that all applicants should undertake a period of physiotherapy clinical experience with a chartered physiotherapist. The website provides helpful information on how to achieve this (www.brunel.ac.uk/courses/ug/cdata/p/ physiotherapy bsc/full details).

Although work-shadowing physiotherapists in specialist areas such as sports clinics or private practices is useful experience it is generally not enough, and applicants without some contact with NHS hospitals are likely to find it hard to get an interview or an offer. If you are very lucky (and very determined) you may be able to get a paid job in an NHS hospital as a physiotherapy assistant. However, because of school or college commitments, this is usually only possible during a gap year. It is more likely that you will have to settle for an unpaid volunteer position either on a part-time basis (at weekends or in the evenings) or for a short period of time in the school holidays. If you are unable to arrange either of these you should try to shadow a physiotherapist for a day or two, and supplement this with a volunteer job in another caring environment such as an old people's home, a hospice, or the children's ward of your local hospital.

Whilst there are no rules about the minimum length of time that you should spend doing work experience, volunteer work or work-shadowing, as a general rule the candidates who can demonstrate commitment by doing something on a regular basis throughout the year or who have spent at least two weeks in a hospital environment are likely to be in the strongest position. Some schools operate schemes where they arrange this for you. This saves you the hard work of contacting hospitals or clinics, but the disadvantage is that you will be unable to impress the selectors with your dynamism and determination because you will not be able to say '*I arranged my work experience myself.*'

'Get as much experience as you can – it doesn't just have to be as a physio assistant. Be determined: there is always a way to get in if you really want to.'

Katherine, University of Hertfordshire

If your school does not operate such a scheme you have two options: to use any contacts that your family or friends have, or to approach local hospitals. To do this you need to get the names and addresses of local hospitals with physiotherapy departments and physiotherapy clinics from the telephone directory. You can also find lists of physiotherapists on the internet. One such site is www.therapy-world.co.uk/physio.htm. You should send an e-mail, and include the name of a referee, someone who can vouch for your interest in physiotherapy as well as for your reliability. Your careers teacher, housemaster/-mistress or form teacher would be ideal. An example of a suitable e-mail is given below.

As well as helping you to decide whether you are serious about physiotherapy and adding weight to your application, work experience is useful because you may be able to get one of the people you work with to give you a reference, which you could send in support of your UCAS application or produce at your interview.

From: Lucy Johnson
To: volunteers@melchesterhospital.org
Subject: Volunteer work

Dear Sir/Madam

I am in the first year of my A level studies, and I am interested in a career in physiotherapy. In order to find out more about physio-therapy I would like to work as a volunteer in the physiotherapy department. I would be able to work on Wednesday afternoons, Saturday afternoons and all day Sunday for the rest of this year. I would be extremely grateful if you would be prepared to meet me, in order to discuss whether it would be possible for me to spend some time at Melchester General Hospital.

If you require a reference, please contact my careers teacher. His name and address are:

Mr N Townson
Head of Careers
Melchester High School
Melchester
MC1 2CD

I look forward to hearing from you.

Yours sincerely

Lucy Johnson

Things to look out for during work experience

The variety of treatments available to patients

Make sure that you know what you are observing. Ask the physiotherapist or nurse for the technical names of the procedures that you see, and for information on the techniques and equipment used. Ask about the advantages and disadvantages of different types of treatments, and in what situations they are used. Keep a diary of what you saw on a day-to-day basis so that you can use it to revise from before an interview. There are a number of websites that provide detailed information on medical conditions and treatments, and you could add further detail to your diary using one of these. The addresses are at the end of the book.

Working as a physiotherapist

Ask the physiotherapist about his/her life. Find out about the hours, how much physiotherapists are paid, the demands of the job and the career options open to physiotherapists. Find out what the physiotherapists like about the job, and what they dislike.

Case Study

Adam first thought of physiotherapy as a possible career when he realised that he was never going to play cricket for England. 'It was never a realistic option because I was never very good at cricket, but I loved sport and I wanted to be involved in it. By the time I was 13 I realised that, if I couldn't make the school team, I certainly wouldn't get a call from England!'

'I got two A grades at GCSE, and the rest were Bs and Cs. I decided to take Biology, Economics and Sports Science for A level, and Physics as an AS level. I found them hard but I knew that I needed BBB to get into Nottingham, my first choice. Someone at school told me that I had to get work experience so I arranged to shadow the physiotherapist at my local football team for three days. Just before I applied I went to an open day and was told that I would probably be rejected because my work experience was insufficient. My form teacher's wife worked at a hospital nearby so she was able to get me into the physiotherapy department there as an assistant very quickly. If I hadn't been to the open day, and been lucky that I had a contact in an NHS physiotherapy department, I wouldn't even have been interviewed.'

Adam's interviews concentrated on his work experience: 'They really probed me about what being a physiotherapist is really like – not just what I did, but what it is like working as a physiotherapist day in and day out, so I'm glad I did it'. Adam received two offers from his four physiotherapy choices. He was not confident about the grades he was going to get, so he put down two other choices – sports science and sports management – where the grade requirements were lower. The work experience convinced him that he desperately wanted to become a physiotherapist. 'I didn't really know what physiotherapy was about, even though I had applied to study it, before I did my work experience. I thought that it was a glamorous job where you worked with sportsmen, got to see sport for free, and spent most of the day chatting about sport. The spell in the hospital showed me what it really entails. Dealing with stroke victims, or old people who don't know what is happening to them, is not easy. You need lots of patience and to really want to make a difference to them. I will probably end up working in a sport-related environment, but I am more open-minded now than I was before.' Adam achieved ABB, higher than the grades that he needed, and is now in his first year at Nottingham.

Tips for work experience

- Dress as the physiotherapists dress: be clean, tidy and reasonably formal
- Offer to help the physiotherapist or the nurses with routine tasks
- Show an interest in all that is going on around you.

Choice of universities

Once you have completed your work experience, and are sure that you want to be a physiotherapist, you need to research your choice of university. There are various factors that you should take into account:

- The type of course
- The entrance requirements (see page 53)
- Location
- Whether you would be taught alongside students on other healthcare courses such as radiology, nursing, occupational therapy or podiatry.

  'My mother worked as an occupational therapist and so I was able to gain extended experience in four major hospitals in the London area. This was absolutely invaluable to me in showing me I wanted to study physiotherapy. This experience was divided between working in mental health and working in the community in order to get a real feeling for getting information across and working as part of a team.'

  Trevor, Bristol UWE

The next step is to get hold of the prospectuses. If your school does not have spare copies telephone the universities, which will send you copies free of charge. Most universities have very informative websites that carry extra information on admissions policies. Once you have narrowed down the number of universities to, say, seven or eight, you should try to visit them in order to get a better idea of what studying there would be like. Your school careers department will have details of open days (or you could telephone the universities directly), and some universities will arrange for you to be shown around at other times of the year as well. Don't simply select your universities because someone tells you that they have good reputations or that they are easier to get into, because you will be spending the next three or four years of your life at one of them, and if you do not like the place you are unlikely to last the course.

Apart from talking to current or former physiotherapy students or careers advisers, there are a number of other sources of information. *The Guardian* newspaper publishes its own league table of universities, ranked by a total score that combines the university's teaching assessment, a 'value-added' score based on the class of degree obtained compared to A level (or equivalent) grades, spending on facilities and materials, student/staff ratio, job prospects and entrance requirements. *The Times* also compiles its own table. The tables can be found at http://education.guardian.co.uk/universityguide and www.timesonline.co.uk. Of course, league tables only tell you a small part of the whole story, and anyone who makes their choices solely on this basis without visiting the universities or reading the prospectuses is taking a serious risk.

■ Academic requirements

In addition to the grades required at A level and AS level, all of the universities specify the minimum grades that they require at GCSE. This varies from university to university, but it is unlikely that you will be considered unless you have at least five or six GCSEs, including science, English and mathematics, taken at one sitting and at B grade or above. If your grades fall below these requirements you need to get your referee to comment on them, either to explain why you underperformed (illness, family disruption etc) or why they expect your A level performance to be better than your GCSE grades indicate.

Students following the A level system should also work hard to ensure that they gain good grades at AS level. Remember that how well you do is important from the start, since not only do AS grades appear on the form but many universities and medical schools will specify minimum grades needed, and may even ask for module breakdowns. Even those that do not have an explicit AS grade requirement will consciously or unconsciously use them as an indicator of your likely A level grades.

Imagine the situation: the selector has one more interview slot to fill, and has the choice between two students with identical work experience, GCSE results and A level predictions; however, one has scored DDDD at AS level, and the other achieved AAAA. Who do you think will get the interview?

The other thing to bear in mind is that a score of DDDD is unlikely to lead to BBB at A level since an AS contributes 50% of the total A level marks, and so the selectors may doubt that the predicted grades are achievable. What this will do is give admissions tutors more to go on than GCSE grades and A level predictions alone, since the AS grades will be published in the August preceding your application and can feature on your UCAS application. It is possible that most universities will specify a minimum AS level requirement for applicants. For the student, this means that the first year of A levels is as important as the second, and the days of the lower sixth being seen as a relaxed year are over.

The importance of the AS levels cannot be understated:

- As the AS scores contribute half of the marks that make up the A level, you should try to resit any weak AS units in the second year of your A levels. This can be done in January or June.
- Coursework units can make a big difference to the final grade – make sure that you are fully aware of the examinations boards' requirements before submitting coursework.
- An understanding of a subject does not mean that you will gain a high grade at AS or A level, as the examiners have very specific requirements. Specimen mark schemes can be found on the examination boards' websites. See page 56 for details.
- Although the details are still to be finalised, it is likely that the universities you apply to will have direct access to all of your AS results (not just the overall grade or even the grade on each paper, but the mark for each paper) from this year.

Entrance requirements vary from university to university, but a 'standard' offer might ask for a minimum of 300 points from 21 units, to include three 6-unit awards or equivalent. The offer would probably specify that biology must be studied to A2 level, along with one other science. This would be satisfied by a student who gained BBC at A level (6-unit awards) and E at AS level (3-unit award). You should also check the university prospectuses for details of A level and AS level requirements. Some universities, for example, specify that they require one of the AS subjects to be an art or humanity, rather than all science/mathematics.

■ Your choices

There are five spaces in the UCAS application, all of which may be used for physiotherapy courses. (In contrast, students applying for medicine, dentistry or veterinary science may only use four of their five choices on these courses.) You do not have to fill all five spaces with physiotherapy courses. You are allowed to apply for a mixture of physiotherapy courses and non-physiotherapy courses, or to leave spaces blank.

If you are worried that you might not be offered a place to study physio-therapy and you would consider other courses, you might want to put down four physiotherapy courses and one other course. The one non-physiotherapy course should be related to physiotherapy, either directly (occupational therapy, podiatry) or in a related discipline such as human biology, physiology, radiology or nursing. You should not enter fewer than four physiotherapy courses in the application because if you do you are unlikely to convince the selectors that you are genuinely committed.

Whatever you do, do not put down medicine or veterinary science as your other choices, because not only will the university or veterinary school reject you, but it will be obvious to the selectors that you are not committed to physiotherapy. If you decide that you would be happy to accept an alternative to physiotherapy if you are unsuccessful, by all means choose another course as long as you feel able to justify the choice at interview. However, our advice is to apply only to physio-therapy courses because:

- It demonstrates to the selectors that you are committed to becoming a physiotherapist.
- You do not run the risk of feeling obliged to accept a place on a course that at heart you do not wish to take. If you are unsuccessful in your initial application for physiotherapy you might be able to gain a place through Clearing, if you accept no alternative offers.
- The more places you apply to, the more chances you are giving yourself.

Once you have made your final choices make sure that you have entered the details into the application correctly. More advice on this can be found in the MPW guide *How to Complete Your UCAS Application*.

■ Personal statement

The personal statement is your chance to show the selectors that:

- You have thought about why you want to be a physiotherapist
- You have investigated the profession
- You would suit the methods of study and lifesyle at their university.

Your UCAS application will be made on-line using the 'apply' system on the UCAS website (www.ucas.com). If you are studying at a school or college, you will be given a 'buzzword' to allow you to apply through them, but individuals can also apply using the on-line system.

The personal statement is your opportunity to demonstrate to the selectors that you have not only researched physiotherapy thoroughly, but also have the right personal qualities to succeed as a physio therapist. Do not be tempted to use overly formal or long-winded English. Read through a draft of your statement, and ask yourself the question '*Does it sound like me?*' If not, rewrite it. Avoid phrases such as '*I was fortunate enough to be able to shadow a physiotherapist ...*' when you really mean '*I shadowed a physiotherapist ...*' or '*I arranged to shadow a physiotherapist ...*'

Why physiotherapy?

A high proportion of UCAS applications contain the phrase '*From an early age I have wanted to be a physiotherapist because it is the only career that combines my love of science with the chance to work with people.*' Not only do admissions tutors get bored with reading this, but it is also clearly untrue: if you think about it, there are many careers that combine science and people, including teaching, pharmacy, dentistry and nursing. However, the basic ideas behind this sentence may well apply to you. If so, you need to personalise it. You could mention an incident that first got you interested in physiotherapy – a visit to a physio-therapist, a conversation with a family friend or a lecture at school, for instance. You could write about your interest in human biology, or a biology project that you undertook when you were younger, to illustrate your interest in science, and you could give examples of how you like to work with others. The important thing is to back up your initial interest in physiotherapy with your efforts to investigate the career.

What have you done to investigate physiotherapy?

This is where you describe your work experience. It is important to demonstrate that you gained something from the work experience, and that it has given you an insight into the profession. You should give an indication of the length of time that you spent at each work placement, what treatments you observed, and your impressions of physiotherapy. You could comment on what aspects of physiotherapy attract you, what you found interesting, or something that surprised you. It is not enough to give details of where you worked and what you saw: the selectors will be asking themselves what you learnt from the experience.

Here is an example of a description of a student's work experience that would not have impressed the selectors:

> *I spent three days at my local hospital's physiotherapy ward. I saw some patients having ultrasounds, and a man who went in the hydrotherapy pool. It was very interesting.*

The next example would have been much more convincing because it is clear that the student was interested in what was happening.

During my three weeks at Melchester General Hospital I was able to shadow two physiotherapists. I watched a range of treatments including ultrasound and exercise in the hydrotherapy pool. I was particularly interested in the ultrasound treatment because I had only ever seen it used for diagnosis. In the cases that I saw during my work experience it was used to stimulate healing in muscle tissue that had been damaged in an accident. Most of the patients that I saw receiving treatment were elderly. I was able to spend some time with a man who had suffered a stroke and had limited use of his hands. The physiotherapist worked with him on a series of repetitive exercises to try to get him to be able to perform simple tasks. I was also able to see the importance of teamwork because the physiotherapist worked alongside a speech therapist as the man had also lost the ability to communicate effectively.

With luck, the selectors may pick up on this at interview, and ask questions about the methods that the physiotherapists used, and the student could then bring in knowledge of ultrasound (having investigated it following his/her work experience). This student would also have gained extra credit with the admissions tutors for having arranged lengthier work experience.

Personal qualities

As a physiotherapist you will be working with others throughout your career. To qualify as a physiotherapist you will study alongside maybe 30 others in your year, for three years. The person reading your UCAS application has to decide two things: whether you have the right personal qualities to become a successful physiotherapist, and whether you will cope with and contribute to university life. To be a successful physiotherapist you need to be able to relate to other people; to survive and enjoy university you need to be able to get on with a wide range of people too. Unlike school life, where many of the activities are organised and arranged by the teachers, almost all of the social activities at university are instigated and organised by the students. For this reason the selectors are looking for people who have the enthusiasm and ability to motivate others, and are prepared to give up their own time to arrange sporting, dramatic, musical or social activities.

'I didn't really know what physiotherapy was about, even though I had applied to study it, before I did my work experience. I thought that it was a glamorous job where you worked with sportsmen, got to see sport for free, and spent most of the day chatting about sport. The spell in hospital showed me what it really entails. Dealing with stroke victims, or old people who don't know what is

happening to them, is not easy. You need lots of patience and to really want to make a difference to them.'

Adam, Nottingham University

A sample personal statement

Why physiotherapy?

I first became interested in becoming a physiotherapist following treatment for a knee injury. This interest was confirmed after attending a seminar given to our school Science Society on biomechanics, and by undertaking several work experience placements. In my local hospital I worked alongside physiotherapists on a neurological rehabilitation ward and was able to observe hydrotherapy treatment and also the treatment of children with cystic fibrosis. I have been helping with a wide range of exercise programmes both in and out of the hydro-therapy pool, and have benefited from the training on subjects that are relevant to children. I have also been involved in teaching swimming to children with learning disabilities and visiting elderly people. This range of experience has helped me to understand the differing demands placed on therapists, the importance of mutual trust and teamwork, and the place of physiotherapy within healthcare.

I have a part time job in my local supermarket dealing with customer enquiries. I found this stressful at first because almost everyone I had to deal with wanted to complain about something! But I soon learnt how to calm them down and to help them to sort out their problems by remaining calm and polite and by listening to what they had to say. I think that this has helped me in my voluntary work as well.

I chose Physics and Sociology at A level, alongside Biology, because they will help me when I study Physiotherapy at university. Physics helps me to develop my problem-solving skills as well as under-standing of the mechanics of movement; and Sociology deals with important issues such as health and illness.

Activities and responsibilities

I participate in many sports, am captain of the school 1st VII netball team and have also played for the 1st XI hockey team. I enjoy textiles and have made several rugs and items of clothing. I like photography, particularly the work of Ansell Adams, who photographed landscapes, and his work has inspired me to go to a number of national parks to take pictures. I go to the cinema and theatre as often as I can and I like music. I have taken grade 7 clarinet and am learning the guitar, which I play badly in a band that I formed with some friends. We have yet to play in public! For my gap year I have arranged to spend six months working in a school for children with serious physical disabilities, and I will then travel with friends to India, Thailand and Vietnam.

How, then, does the person reading your personal statement know whether you have the qualities that they are looking for? They will expect to read about some of the following:

- Participation in team events
- Involvement in school plays or concerts
- Positions of responsibility
- Work in the local community
- Part-time or holiday jobs
- Charity work.

The selectors will be aware that some schools offer more in the way of activities and responsibilities than others, and they will make allowances for this. You don't have to have been on a school expedition to India or to be Head Girl to be considered, but you need to be able to demonstrate that you have taken the best possible advantage of what is on offer. The selectors will be aware of the type of school or college that you have come from (there is a box on the back of the UCAS application that your referee fills in) and, consequently, the opportunities that are open to you. What they are looking for is that you have grasped these opportunities.

■ The reference

As well as your GCSE results and your personal statement, the selectors will take your reference into account. This is where your head, housemaster/-mistress or head of sixth form writes about what an outstanding person you are, the life and soul of the school; how you are on target for three A grades at A level; and why you will become an outstanding physiotherapist. For him or her to say this, of course, it has to be true. The referee is expected to be as honest as possible, and to try to accurately assess your character and potential. You may believe that you have all of the qualities, academic and personal, necessary in a physiotherapist, but unless you have demonstrated these to your teachers they will be unable to support your application. Ideally your efforts to impress them will have begun at the start of the sixth form (or before): you will have become involved in school activities, you will have been working hard at your studies and you will be popular with students and teachers alike. However, it is never too late, and some people mature later than others, so if this does not sound like you, start to make efforts to impress the people who will contribute to your reference.

As part of the reference your referee will need to predict the grades that you are likely to achieve. As you will see from the table on pages 53–4 most universities ask for at least BBB. If you are predicted lower than this it is unlikely that you will be considered. Talk to your teachers and find out whether you are on target for these grades. If not, you need to a) work harder or more effectively – and make sure that your teachers notice that you are doing so, or b) get some extra help either at school or outside, for instance by taking an Easter revision course, or c) delay submitting your UCAS application until you have your A level results. If you decide on this option make sure that you use your gap year wisely (see below).

When to submit the UCAS application

The closing date for receipt of the application by UCAS is 15 January. Late applications are accepted by UCAS, but the universities are not obliged to consider them, and because of the pressure on places it is unlikely that late applications will be considered. Although you can submit your application any time between the beginning of September and the January deadline (remembering to get it to your referee at least two weeks before the deadline so that he/she has time to prepare the reference), most admissions tutors admit that the earlier the application is submitted the better your chance of being called for interview. Your best bet is to talk to the person who will deal with the application in the summer term of your first year of A levels, and work on your personal statement and choice of universities over the summer holidays so that it is ready to hand in at the start of the September term.

'I chose St George's because it offered early and very good clinical contact and training alongside other healthcare professionals, and because they were the most helpful prior to submitting my application. I was really glad that I spent a long time studying the prospectuses, looking at websites, talking to physiotherapy students, coaches, admissions tutors and advisors at my college because I then was able to make a very informed decision about the most suitable course for me.'

Alice, St George's

Deferred entry

Most admissions tutors are happy to consider students who take a gap year, and many encourage it. However, if you are considering this, you need to make sure that you are going to use the time constructively. A year spent watching daytime TV is not going to impress anybody, whereas independent travelling, charity or voluntary work either at home or abroad, work experience or a responsible job will all indicate that you have used the time to develop independence and maturity. Above all, make sure that whatever you do with the year involves regular contact with other people.

You can either apply for deferred entry when you submit your UCAS application, in which case you need to outline your plans in your personal statement, or apply in September following the publication of your A level results. If you expect to be predicted the right grades, and the feedback from your school or college is that you will be given a good reference, you should apply for deferred entry; but if you are advised by your referee that you are unlikely to be considered you should give yourself more time to work on your referees by waiting until you have your A level results.

The number of deferred places varies between universities, and from year to year. As an example, Nottingham University made nine deferred offers for 2005 entry.

■ What happens next?

When the staff at UCAS receive your application they will send you an acknowledgement. About two weeks later you will receive a statement of entry, which lists all of your choices. Check this carefully – make sure that the universities and course codes are correct, and that your name and address are also correct. Remember also to inform UCAS if you change address.

The next correspondence you will receive, if you are lucky, is likely to be from the universities, asking you to attend an interview. Don't be alarmed if you do not hear anything soon after UCAS has sent you your statement of entry. Some universities interview on a first come, first served basis whilst others wait until all applications are in before deciding whom to interview. It is not uncommon for students to hear nothing until after Christmas.

If you are unlucky you will receive a slip from UCAS telling you that you have been rejected by one or more of the universities. Don't despair: you may hear better news from another of the places that you applied to. Even if you get five rejections the worst thing that you can do is give up and decide that it is no longer worth working hard. On the contrary, if this does happen, you should become even more determined to gain high grades so that you can apply either through Clearing, or the following year. The process of making Clearing applications is discussed on pages 33–4.

■ Checklist

- At least two weeks' NHS work-shadowing?
- Voluntary work?
- Right GCSE subjects and grades?
- Right A level subjects?
- On target for required grades?
- Looked at all the universities' prospectuses?

- Open days?
- Minimum of four physiotherapy choices in the UCAS application?
- Personal statement demonstrates commitment, research, personal qualities, communication skills and manual dexterity?

For the latest news on physiotherapy and physiotherapy courses, go to www.mpw.co.uk/getintomed

02 Getting an offer

If the selectors like the picture that the UCAS application has painted of you they will call you for interview. The purpose of the interview is to allow them to see whether this picture is an accurate one, and to investigate whether you have a genuine interest in physiotherapy. The interviewers will generally ask you three types of question:

1| Those designed to relax you so that they can assess your communication skills
2| Those designed to investigate your interest and suitability for physiotherapy
3| Those designed to get a clearer picture of your personal qualities.

■ Interview questions

Questions to get you relaxed

How was your journey here today?

The interviewers are not really interested in the details of your travels. Do not be tempted to give them a minute-by-minute account of your bus journey ('... and then we waited for six minutes at the roadworks on Corporation Street ...'), but also do not simply say 'OK'. Say something like 'It was fine, thank you. The train journey took about two hours, which gave me the chance to catch up on some reading'. With a bit of luck they will ask you what you read, which gives you the chance to talk about a book, newspaper article or an item in New Scientist.

I am interested to know why you decided to apply to Melchester.

Another variation on this might be 'How did you narrow your choice down to five universities?' The panel will be looking for evidence of research, and that your reasons are based on informed judgement. Probably the best possible answer would start with 'I came to your open day ...' because you can then proceed to tell them why you like their university so much, what impressed you about the course and facilities and how the atmosphere of the place would particularly suit you. Even if you are unable to attend open days try to arrange a formal or informal visit before you are interviewed so that you can show that you are aware of the environment, both academic and physical, and that you like the place. If you know people who are at the university or on the course, so much the better. You should also know about the course structure. On page 53 there is an overview of the differences and similarities between courses, and the prospectus will give detailed information. Given the choice between a candidate who is not only going to make a good physiotherapist, but clearly wants to come to their institution, and another who may have the right qualities but does not seem to care whether it is there or somewhere else that he/she studies, whom do you think the selectors will choose?

Answers to avoid are 'Reputation', unless you know in detail the areas for which the university is highly regarded; 'It's in London, and I don't want to move away from my friends'; 'You take a lot of retake students'; 'My dad says it is easy to get a place here'.

A good answer could be 'I came to an open day last summer, which is why I have applied here. I enjoyed the day, and was impressed by the facilities, and by the comments of the students who showed us around because they seemed so enthusiastic about the course. Also, my cousin studied English at the university and I visited her, and got to sample the atmosphere of the town.'

There are variations on this question. The interviewers may ask you what you know about the course, or about the university. In all cases this is your chance to show the interviewers that you are desperate to come to their university.

A word of warning: do your homework by reading the prospectus and looking at the website. Although on the surface all physiotherapy courses appear to cover broadly the same subjects, there are big differences in how the courses are delivered, and in the opportunities for patient contact, and your interviewers will expect you to know about their course.

Questions about physiotherapy

Why do you want to be a physiotherapist?
The question that all interviewees expect. Given that the interviewers will be aware that you are expecting the question, they will also expect your answer to be carefully planned. If you look surprised, and say something like 'Um ... well ... I haven't really thought about why ...' you can expect to be rejected. Other answers to avoid are: 'The money'; 'I couldn't get into medicine'; 'I want to help people'; 'I want to work for Arsenal'.

Many students are worried that they will sound insincere when they answer this question. The way to avoid this is to try to bring in reasons that are personal to you, for instance an incident that started your interest (perhaps a visit to a physiotherapist), or an aspect of your work experience that particularly fascinated you. The important thing is to try to express clearly what interested you rather than try to generalise your answers. Rather than say 'Physiotherapy combines science, working with people and the chance to have control over your career' – which says little about you, tell the interviewers about the way that your interest progressed. Here is an example of a good answer:

> Although it seemed strange to my friends, I used to enjoy going with my grandfather to a physiotherapist when he had difficulty in walking due to arthritis. This was because the physiotherapist explained things very clearly and patiently, and I was interested in what was happening around me. My favourite subject is biology, particularly the anatomy side of it, and I always wanted to do something that involved this. When I was thinking about my career I arranged to shadow another physiotherapist, and the more time I spent at the hospital the more I realised that this would really suit me. This also gave me the chance to find out about what being a physiotherapist is really like. The things about physiotherapy that I particularly enjoy are …

WARNING: Do not learn this passage and repeat it at your interview. Ensure that your answer is not only personal to you, but also honest.

With luck, the interviewers will pick up on something that you said about work experience, and ask you more questions about this.

Since 'Why do you want to be a physiotherapist?' is such an obvious question, interviewers often try to find out the information in different ways. Expect questions such as 'When did your interest in physio-therapy start?', or 'What was it about your work experience that finally convinced you that physiotherapy was for you?'

I see that you spent two weeks with your physiotherapist. Was there anything that surprised you?

Variations on this question could include 'Was there anything that partic-ularly interested you?', 'Was there anything you found off-putting?' or simply 'Tell me about your work experience'. What these questions really mean is 'Are you able to show us that you were interested in what was happening during your work experience?' Returning to the original question, answering either 'Yes' or 'No' without explanation will not gain you many marks. Similarly, saying 'Yes, I was surprised by the number of patients who seemed very scared' says nothing about your awareness of the physiotherapist's approach to his/her patients. However, answering 'Yes, I was surprised by the number of patients who seemed very scared. What struck me, however, was the way in which the physiotherapist dealt with each patient as an individual, sometimes being sympathetic, sometimes explaining things in great detail and sometimes using humour to relax them. For instance ...' shows that you were interested enough to be aware of more than the most obvious things. Sentences that start with 'For example ...' and 'For instance ...' are particularly important as they allow you to demonstrate your interest. In order to be able to give examples you should keep a diary of things that you saw during your work experience so that you do not forget. You should read through this before your interview, as if you were revising for an examination.

I see that you try to keep up to date with developments in physiotherapy. Can you tell me about something that you have read about recently?

If you are interested in making physiotherapy your career the selectors will expect you to be interested enough in the subject to want to read about it. Good sources of information are the Chartered Society of Physiotherapy's website and others (addresses are given at the end of the book), *New Scientist* and the national newspapers. You should get into the habit of looking at a broadsheet newspaper every day to see if there are any medically or physiotherapy-related stories. Note that the question uses the word recently: recent does not mean an article you read two years ago – keep up to date. You could, for instance, say *'There was a recent report that sportspeople risk injury from air-filled training shoes. There was a survey of basketball players which showed that they were four times more likely to suffer ankle injuries if they were wearing trainers with soles that contained air pockets.'*

During your work experience, you had the chance to discuss physiotherapy with physiotherapists. What do you know about career opportunities and pay for physiotherapists?

You must make sure that you do some research on career paths by asking questions about this when you meet physiotherapists. Most physiotherapists work in the NHS, but there are many other options. On page 1 we described many of the types of work undertaken by physiotherapists. Most physiotherapists end up specialising in one or more particular areas – in most cases as a result of an interest that grew during their training. The best answer to a question like this is to describe the career paths of physiotherapists you have met and worked with, as this will allow you to highlight your own work experience.

What qualities should a physiotherapist possess?

These have been discussed on page 14. However, don't simply list them. The question has not been asked because the interviewer is puzzled about what these qualities are; it has been asked to give you a chance to show a) that you are aware of them, and b) that you possess them. The best way to answer this is to use phrases such as '*During my work experience at the Melchester Physiotherapy Clinic I was able to observe/talk to the physiotherapist, and I became aware that ...*', or '*Communication is very important. For instance, when I was shadowing my physiotherapist, there was a patient who ...*' Try always to relate these general questions to your own experiences.

Physiotherapy requires high levels of physical fitness and manual dexterity. Do you possess these?

Manual manipulation of a patient's limbs requires a fair degree of fitness and strength, and as a physiotherapist you will need to be able to help to lift and lower patients. If you have trouble picking up a coffee cup without breathing heavily for the next ten minutes physiotherapy may not be the best career for you. The interviewers will need to be reassured that you are able to work in a physically demanding environment, and also that you have the manual dexterity necessary to perform sometimes intricate tasks. Try to anticipate this question by preparing an answer which demonstrates that you have these qualities. Sport is always a good indicator of fitness and coordination, but you could also mention situations that you encountered during your work experience, demanding tasks that you perform as part of a weekend job, expeditions that you have been on at school as part of the Duke of Edinburgh Award, or a hobby such as DIY.

WARNING: Do not lie about the example you describe. An admissions tutor I talked to recounted the story of an applicant who wrote in the UCAS application that he worked for a local Riding for the Disabled scheme. However, the previous interview had been with someone from the same town who had explained that there was no such sceme in the area, which is why she could not carry on doing this when she moved into the area. He was found out, and rejected.

Questions to find out about what sort of person you are

What do you do to relax?

Don't say '*Watch TV*' or '*Go to the pub*'. Mention something that involves working or communicating with others, for instance sport or music. Use the question to demonstrate that you possess the qualities required in a physiotherapist. However, don't make your answer so insincere that the interviewers realise that you are trying to impress them. Saying '*I relax most effectively when I go to the local physiotherapy clinic to shadow the physiotherapist*' will not convince them.

How do you cope with stress?

Physiotherapy can be a stressful occupation. Physiotherapists have to deal with difficult people, those who are scared and those who react badly when in a physiotherapy ward. For many people, physiotherapy can be painful and distressing and patients are not always cooperative, or even aware of why they are receiving treatment. In these circumstances the physiotherapist cannot panic, but must remain calm and rational. The interviewers will want to make a judgement as to whether you will be able to cope with the demands of the job.

Having been through it themselves, it is unlikely that they will regard school examinations as being particularly stressful. Hard work, yes, but not as stressful as training to be a physiotherapist or practising as a physiotherapist. What they are looking for are answers that demonstrate your calmness and composure when dealing with others. You could relate it to your work experience, or your Saturday job. Dealing with a queue of angry and impatient customers demanding to know why their cheeseburgers are not ready can be difficult. Other areas that can provide evidence of stress management are school expeditions, public speaking, or positions of responsibility at school or outside.

I see that you enjoy reading. What is the most recent book that you have read?

The question might be about the cinema or theatre, but the point of it is the same: to get you talking about something that interests you. Although it may sound obvious, if you have written that you enjoy reading in your UCAS application make sure that you have actually read something recently. Admissions tutors will be able to tell you stories about interviewees who look at them with absolute amazement when they are asked about books, despite it featuring in the personal statement. Answers such as '*Well … I haven't had much time recently, but … let me see … I read* Elle *last month, and … oh yes … I had to read Jane Eyre for my English GCSE*' will do your chances no good at all. By all means put down that you like reading, but make sure that you have read an interesting novel in the period leading up to the interview, and be prepared to discuss it.

■ How to succeed in your interview

You should prepare for an interview as if you are preparing for an examination. This involves revision of your work experience diary so that you can recount details of your time with physiotherapists, revision of the newspaper, website and *New Scientist* articles that you have saved and revision of all of the things that you have mentioned on your personal statement. When you are preparing for your A levels you sit a mock examination so that the real thing does not come as a total surprise;

when you are preparing for an interview have a mock interview so that you can get some feedback on your answers. Your school may be able to help you. If not, independent sixth-form colleges usually provide a mock interview service. Friends of your parents may also be able to help. If possible, video your mock interview so that you are aware of the way you come across in an interview situation. There is a list of practice interview questions below.

■ Mock interview questions

1| Why do you want to be a physiotherapist?
2| What have you done to investigate physiotherapy?
3| Why does physiotherapy interest you more than medicine/nursing/ radiography?
4| What are the ideal qualities that a physiotherapist should possess?
5| Do you possess these qualities?
6| Give me an example of how you cope with stress.
7| Why did you apply to this university?
8| Did you come to our open day?
9| During your work experience, did anything surprise you?
10| During your work experience, did anything shock you?
11| Was the physiotherapist you shadowed good at communicating with his/her patients?
12| Tell me about preventive physiotherapy.
13| What is occupational therapy?
14| What is repetitive strain injury?
15| What is cystic fibrosis/a stroke/arthritis?
16| What is hydrotherapy?
17| What is ultrasound and how is it used?
18| Is exercise always good for you?
19| How much do NHS physiotherapists earn?
20| Have you read any articles about physiotherapy recently?
21| What advances can we expect in physiotherapy technology/ treatment in the future?
22| What have you done to demonstrate your commitment to the community?
23| What would you contribute to this university?
24| What are your best/worst qualities?
25| What was the last novel you read? What did you think of it?
26| What was the last play/film you saw? What did you think of it?
27| What do you do to relax?
28| What is your favourite A level subject?
29| What grades do you expect to gain in your A levels?
30| What precautions need to be taken with patients who are HIV positive?
31| How does teamwork apply to the role of a physiotherapist?
32| What branch of physiotherapy interests you the most, and why?

33| What is the role of a physiotherapist in a hospital?

34| Why are communication skills important for physiotherapists?

35| What have you done that demonstrates your communication skills?

36| What have you done that demonstrates your leadership skills?

37| What have you done that demonstrates your ability to cope in a stressful situation?

38| Why is a knowledge of physics helpful in physiotherapy?

39| What are the particular difficulties that animal physiotherapists encounter?

40| How did you organise your work experience?

41| Why are you taking a gap year?

> `My interviews concentrated on my work experience. They really probed me about what being a physiotherapist is really like – not just what I did, but what it is like working as a physiotherapist day in and day ouut, so I'm glad I did it.'
>
> **Adam Nottingham University**

Appearance and body language are important. The impression you create can be very influential. Remember that if the interviewers cannot picture you as a physiotherapist in future years they are unlikely to offer you a place.

Body language

- Maintain eye contact with the interviewers.
- Direct most of what you are saying to the person who asked you the question, but occasionally look around at the others on the panel.
- Sit up straight, but adopt a position that you feel comfortable in.
- Don't wave your hands around too much, but don't keep them gripped together to stop them moving. Fold them across your lap, or rest them on the arms of the chair.

Speech

- Talk slowly and clearly.
- Don't use slang.
- Avoid saying 'erm ...', 'you know', 'sort of'.
- Say hello at the start of the interview, and thank you and goodbye at the end.

Dress and appearance

- Wear clothes that show you have made an effort for the interview. You do not have to wear a business suit, but a jacket and tie (men) or a skirt and blouse (women) are appropriate.
- Make sure that you are clean and tidy.

- If appropriate, shave before the interview (but avoid overpowering aftershave).
- Clean your nails and shoes.
- Wash your hair.
- Avoid (visible) piercings, earrings (men), jeans and trainers.

At the end of the interview

You may be given the opportunity to ask a question at the end of the interview. Bear in mind that the interviews are carefully timed, and that your attempts to impress the panel with 'clever' questions may do quite the opposite. The golden rule is: only ask a question if you are genuinely interested in the answer (which, of course, you were unable to find during your careful reading of the prospectus).

Questions to avoid

- *'What is the structure of the first year of the course?'*
- *'Will I be able to live in a hall of residence?'*
- *'When will I first have contact with patients?'*

As well as being boring questions, the answers to these will be available in the prospectus. You have obviously not done any serious research.

Questions you could ask

- *'I haven't studied Physics AS level. Should I go through some physics textbooks before the start of the course?'*
- This shows that you are keen, and that you want to make sure that you can cope with the course. It will give the selectors a chance to talk about the extra course they offer for non-physicists.
- *'Do you think I should try to get more work experience before the start of the course?'*

  Again, an indication of your keenness.

- *'Earlier, I couldn't answer the question you asked me on ultrasound. What is the answer?'*
- Something that you genuinely might want to know.
- *'How soon will you let me know if I have been successful or not?'*

  Something you really want to know.

REMEMBER: If in doubt, don't ask a question. End by saying 'All of my questions have been answered by the prospectus and the students who showed me around the university. Thank you very much for an interesting day.' Smile, shake hands (if appropriate – if you are being interviewed by a panel of five, who are all sitting at the other end of a long table, then don't!) and say goodbye.

■ Structuring the interview

The selectors will have a set of questions that they may ask, designed to assess your suitability and commitment. If you answer '*Yes*' or '*No*' to most questions, or reply only in monosyllables, they will fire more and more questions at you. If, however, your answers are longer and also contain statements that interest them, they are more likely to pick up on these, and you are, effectively, directing the interview. If you are asked questions that you have prepared for there will be less time for the interviewers to ask you questions that might be more difficult to answer.

For example, at the end of your answer to a question about work experience, you might say '*... and the physiotherapist was able to explain the effect of new technology on physiotherapy.*' The interviewer may then say '*I see. Can you tell me about how technology is changing physiotherapy?*' You can then embark on an answer about ultrasound, for instance. At the end of your explanation you could finish with: '*...of course, ultrasound treatment is often used in conjunction with infrared radiation treatment.*' You may then be asked about situations where this might happen, and so on.

Of course this does not always work, but you would be very unlucky not to have at least one of these 'signposts' that you placed in front of them followed.

■ How you are selected

During the interview the panel will be assessing you in various categories. Whether or not the interview appears to be structured the interviewers will be following careful guidelines so that they can compare candidates from different interview sessions. Some panels adopt a conversational style, whereas others are more formal. The scoring system will vary from place to place but, in general, you will be assessed in the following categories:

- Reason for your choice of university
- Academic ability
- Motivation for physiotherapy
- Awareness of physiotherapy issues
- Personal qualities
- Communication skills.

You are likely to be scored in each category, and the university will have a minimum mark that you will have to gain if you are to be made an offer. If you are below this score, but close to it, you may be put on an official or unofficial waiting list. If this happens you may be considered in August, should there be places available.

If you are offered a place you will receive a letter from the university telling you what you need to achieve in your A levels. This is called a Conditional Offer. Post-A level students who have achieved the necessary grades will be given Unconditional Offers. If you are unlucky all you will get is an e-mail from UCAS saying that you have been rejected. If this happens it is not necessarily the end of the road that leads you to a career in physio-therapy. If you are rejected by all of your choices, you can enter the 'UCAS Extra' scheme which allows you to contact other universities. If you still are without a place when the A level results are released in August, you are eligible to apply for vacant places through Clearing.

When UCAS has received replies from all of your choices they will send you a Statement of Offers. You will then have about a month to make up your mind about where you want to go. If you only have one offer you have little choice but to accept it. If you have more than one you have to accept one as your Firm choice, and another (usually a lower offer) as your Insurance choice. If the place where you really want to study makes a lower offer than one of your other choices do not be tempted to choose the lower offer as your Insurance, since you are obliged to go to the university that you have put as your Firm choice if you achieve the grades. Even if you narrowly miss you may still be accepted by your first choice. If you decide that you do not want to go there, once the results are issued, you will have to withdraw from the UCAS system for that year.

For the latest news on physiotherapy and physiotherapy courses, go to www.mpw.co.uk/getintomed

03 Results day

The A level results will arrive at your school on the third Thursday in August. The universities will have received them a few days earlier. You must make sure that you go into school on the day the results are published. Don't wait for the results slip to be posted to you. Get your teachers to tell you the news as soon as possible. If you need to act to secure a place you may have to do so quickly.

The university admissions departments are well organised and efficient, but they are staffed by human beings. If there were extenuating circumstances that could have affected your exam performance and which were brought to their notice in June, it is a good idea to ask them to review the relevant letters shortly before the exam results are published.

If you previously received a Conditional Offer and your grades equal or exceed that offer, congratulations! You can relax and wait for your chosen university to send you joining instructions. One word of warning: you cannot assume that grades of AAC satisfy an ABB offer. This is especially true if the C grade is in Biology.

The following paragraphs take you through the steps necessary to use the UCAS Extra and Clearing systems. They also explain what to do if your grades are disappointing.

■ What to do if you have no offer

If all of the universities that you applied to reject you, you are then eligible to enter a scheme called 'UCAS Extra'. This allows you to apply to other universities, either for physiotherapy or for other courses. You will automatically be sent details by UCAS. UCAS Extra starts in March. If UCAS Extra does not provide you with an offer, you can enter Clearing in August.

These days very few applicants get into university through Clearing. Very few universities have spare places in August and, of those that do, most will choose to allow applicants who hold a Conditional Offer to slip a grade rather than dust off a reserve list of those they interviewed but didn't make an offer to. Still less are they likely to consider applicants who appear out of the blue – however high their grades. That said, it is likely that every summer one or two universities will have enough unfilled places to consider a Clearing-style application.

If you hold, say, AAB but were rejected when you applied through UCAS you need to let the universities know that you are out there. The best way to do this is by e-mail. E-mail addresses and phone numbers are listed in the *UCAS Handbook*. If you live nearby you can always deliver a letter in person, talk to the office staff and hope that your application will stand out from the rest. Set out on this page is a sample e-mail. Don't copy it word for word!

Don't forget that your UCAS referee may be able to help you. Try to persuade him or her to ring the admissions officers on your behalf – he or she will find it easier to get through than you will. If your headteacher is unable/unwilling to ring, then he or she should, at least, e-mail a note in support of your application. It is best if both e-mails arrive at the university at the same time.

If you are applying to a university that did not receive your UCAS application ask your head to e-mail or send a copy of the application. In general it is best to persuade the university to invite you to arrange for the UCAS application to be sent.

If, despite your most strenuous efforts, you are unsuccessful, you need to consider applying again (see page 37). The other alternative is to use the Clearing system to obtain a place on a degree course related to physiotherapy and hope to be accepted on a physiotherapy course after you graduate. This option is described on page 39.

From: Lucy Johnson
To: mdwhyte@melchester.ac.uk
Subject: Physiotherapy places

Dear Miss Whyte

UCAS No 07-123456-8

I have just received my A level results, which were:
Biology B, Chemistry B, English C.
I also have an A grade in AS Photography.

You may remember that I applied to Melchester but was rejected after interview/was rejected without an interview. I am still very keen to study physiotherapy at Melchester and hope that you will consider me for any places that may now be available.

My headteacher supports my application and is faxing you a reference. Should you wish to contact him, the details are: Mr C Harrow, Tel: 0123 456 7891, Fax: 0123 456 7892. I can be contacted at the above address and could attend an interview at short notice.

Lucy Johnson

What to do if you hold an offer but miss the grades

If you have only narrowly missed the required grades (this includes the AAC grade case described above) it is important that you and your referee e-mail the university to put your case before you are rejected. Another sample e-mail follows below.

From: Lucy Johnson
To: mdwhyte@melchester.ac.uk
Subject: A level results

Dear Miss Whyte

UCAS No 07-123456-8

I have just received my A level results, which were:
Biology B, Chemistry B, English C.

I hold a conditional offer from Melchester of ABB and I realise that my grades fall below that offer. Nevertheless, I am still determined to study physiotherapy and I hope you will be able to find a place for me this year.

I would like to remind you that at the time of the exams I was recovering from glandular fever. A medical certificate was sent to you in June by my headteacher.

My headteacher supports my application and is faxing you a reference. Should you wish to contact him, the details are: Mr C Harrow, Tel: 0123 456 7891, Fax: 0123 456 7892. I can be contacted at the above address and could attend an interview at short notice.

Lucy Johnson

If this is unsuccessful you need to consider retaking your A levels and applying again (see page 37). The other alternative is to use the Clearing system to obtain a place on a degree course related to physiotherapy and hope to apply to the physiotherapy course after you graduate. This option is described on page 39.

Retaking your A levels

The grade requirements for retake candidates are often higher than for first timers. You should contact the universities to find out what they require from retake students. Many A levels can be retaken in January, but this depends on the board as well as the subject. The school or college where you will sit the retakes will be able to help you. The timescale for your retake will depend on:

- The grades you obtained first time
- The examination board through which you studied.

If you simply need to improve one subject by one or two grades and can retake the exam on the same syllabus in January then the short retake course is the logical option. If, on the other hand, your grades were DDE and you took your exams through a board that has no mid-year retakes you probably need to spend another year on your retakes. You would find it almost impossible to master syllabus changes in three subjects and achieve an increase of nine or ten grades within the 17 weeks or so that are available for teaching between September and January.

Independent sixth-form colleges provide specialist advice and teaching for students considering A level retakes. Interviews to discuss this are free and carry no obligation to enrol on a course, so it is worth taking the time to talk to their staff before you embark on A level retakes.

■ Re-applying to university

The choice of universities for your UCAS application is going to be narrower than it was the first time round. Don't apply to the universities that discourage retakers unless there really are special, extenuating circumstances to explain your disappointing grades. The following are examples of excuses that would not be regarded by admissions tutors as extenuating circumstances:

> 'I was revising on my dad's yacht and my files got soaked when I accidentally dropped them in the sea.'

> 'I left my bag on the bus the week before the exams, and all of my notes were in it, so I couldn't do any revision.'

> 'We moved house a month before the exams and a removal man trod on my notes, so I couldn't revise properly from them.'

Some reasons are acceptable to even the most fanatical opponents of retake candidates:

■ Your own illness
■ The death or serious illness of a very close relative.

These are just guidelines, and the only safe method of finding out if a university will accept you is to write and ask them. A typical e-mail is set out on page 38. Don't follow it word for word and do take the time to write to several universities before you make your final choice.

Notice that the format of your e-mail should be:

■ Opening paragraph
■ Your exam results – set out clearly, with no omissions
■ Any extenuating circumstances – a brief statement
■ Your retake plan – including the timescale
■ A request for help and advice
■ Closing paragraph.

Make sure that your e-mail is brief, clear and well presented. Even if you go to this trouble, the pressure on universities in the autumn is such that you may receive no more than a standard reply to the effect that, if you apply, your application will be considered.

Apart from the care needed in making the choice of university, the rest of the application procedure is as described in the first part of this book.

From: Lucy Johnson
To: mdwhyte@melchester.ac.uk
Subject: Application for physiotherapy

Dear Miss Whyte

Last year's UCAS No. 07-123456-8

I am writing to ask your advice because I am about to complete my UCAS application and would very much like to apply to Melchester. You may remember that I applied to you last year and received an offer of BBB/was rejected after interview/was rejected without an interview.

I have just received my A level results, which were:
Biology B, Chemistry C, English E.
I was aged 17 years and six months at the time of taking these exams.

I plan to retake Biology in January after a 17-week course and English over a year. If necessary, I will retake Chemistry in the period from January to June. I am confident that I can push these subjects up to ABB grades overall.

What worries me is that I have heard that some universities do not consider retake candidates even when the exams were taken under the age of 18 and relatively high grades were obtained. I am very keen not to waste a slot on my UCAS form (or your time) by applying to departments that will reject me purely because I am retaking.

I am very keen to come to Melchester, and would be extremely grateful for any advice that you can give me.

Lucy Johnson

■ Non-standard applications

So far, this book has been concerned with the 'standard' applicant: the UK resident who is studying at least two science subjects at A level and who is applying from school or who is retaking immediately after disappointing A levels. The main non-standard categories are as follows.

Those who have not studied science A levels

If you decide that you would like to study physiotherapy after having already started on a combination of A levels that does not fit the subject requirements for entry to university, you have three choices.

1| You can spend an extra year studying science A levels at a sixth-form college that offers one-year AS/A2 courses. You should discuss your particular circumstances with prospective colleges in order to select suitable courses. It is worth being aware that only very able students can cover A level Chemistry and Biology in a single year with good results.
2| You can follow a foundation course at a university that will then allow you to study a related degree course afterwards. For details of foundation courses you should contact universities.
3| You can enrol on an Access course which is recognised by the universities you wish to apply to. Each university will have different policies about Access courses – you should contact the physiotherapy departments directly.

Overseas students

The competition for the few places available to non-EU students is fierce and you would be wise to discuss your application informally with the university before submitting it. In general, overseas applicants will find it difficult to gain a place unless they can offer qualifications that are recognised by the universities, such as A levels or the IB.

Information about qualifications can be obtained from British Council offices, British Embassies and the universities that offer physiotherapy courses.

Overseas students are liable for the full cost of tuition. For physiotherapy the fees vary, depending on the university, but will be in the region of £11,000 per year.

Mature students and graduates

Physiotherapy courses are popular with older students, and the universities tend to have a flexible and encouraging approach to students over the age of 21. Approximately 30% of students studying physiotherapy are mature students.

Graduates

An upper second class degree (or higher) along with at least a grade B in A level Biology is normally required. Most universities ask graduates to take a year out between the final year of their first degree course and the start of the physiotherapy course in order to get work experience. This allows them to demonstrate that they are serious about a career in physiotherapy.

Applicants with no suitable academic qualifications

Candidates are likely to be asked to sit at least two A levels, one of which will be Biology, and to achieve B grades or higher. There are also some Access courses that can lead to an offer of a place to study physiotherapy; applicants should liaise with universities to confirm suitability.

The main difficulty facing those who come late to the idea of studying physiotherapy is that they rarely have a scientific background. They face the daunting task of studying science A levels and need very careful counselling before they embark on what will, inevitably, be quite a tough programme. Independent sixth-form colleges provide this counselling as part of their normal interview procedure.

■ Students not studying A levels

As with A levels, entrance requirements will vary from university to university. The information below is given as a guideline only.

- **BTEC Higher National Diploma:** 16 units, mostly biology or life sciences, with merits and distinctions throughout.
- **BTEC National Certificate:** 18 units, mostly biology and life sciences, with merits and distinctions throughout; plus one A level or two AS levels.
- **Advanced Vocational Certificate of Education:** 12 units with science or healthcare-related options, possibly with one A level or two AS levels.
- **Irish Leaving Certificate:** six papers taken at one sitting, at Higher Level, to include at least AABBB, or 400+ points.
- **Scottish Highers:** 300 points, to include two sciences.
- **IB:** 32 points with biology at higher level.

Other qualifications, such as the European Baccalaureate, the French Baccalaureate or Open University qualifications, or the successful completion of a recognised Access course, will usually be considered but this is no guarantee that an offer will be made. You should make contact with university admissions tutors or look on the university websites for advice.

> 'When we interview students, we want to find out two things –
> whether they are really committed to the profession, and whether
> they have the right personality to succeed. For the first of these, it
> is work experience, work experience, work experience that
> matters. For the second, I look for the ability to respond to my
> questions calmly and with structure. I also look at whether they
> have contributed to the life of their school, college or community.'

Admissions tutor

For the latest news on physiotherapy and physiotherapy courses, go to www.mpw.co.uk/getintomed

---

04 Useful information

■ Typical course structure

Whilst all physiotherapy courses contain many common elements there are significant differences in the structure of these courses, in the course content, in the way in which the practical and patient-contact elements are arranged, and in the styles of assessment. You should investigate this thoroughly by reading prospectuses and looking at the physiotherapy departments' websites in order to find out which ones will best suit you.

First year

Underlying theory and practical issues

- Anatomy
- Cardiovascular and respiratory functions
- Communication and clinical skills
- Kinesiology (the mechanics of body movement)
- Musculoskeletal conditions
- Physiology
- Research methods.

Second year

- Neurology
- Pathophysiology
- Clinical education, taking into account social, cultural and economic factors
- Clinical placements.

The second-year course divides the time between academic study and clinical placements. Clinical placements take place in a variety of settings, including hospital wards, physiotherapy outpatients departments and specialised units within hospitals and the community. The clinical placements will focus on areas such as orthopaedics, rehabilitation and community medicine. Chartered Society of Physiotherapy guidelines require a certain number of hours (1000) of clinical practice to be undertaken in order to gain recognition, and the 16 weeks of clinical placement are usually in the order of 30 hours per week.

Third year

The third year will also be split between clinical and academic study – students will usually spend about 20 weeks of the course on clinical placements. Specialist areas of study could include:

- Burns and plastic surgery
- Exercise and sports science
- Learning difficulties
- Mental health
- Neurology
- Neurorehabilitation
- Outpatients
- Paediatrics
- Pain management
- Respiratory medicine.

Elective clinical placement

At the end of the third year there might be an elective clinical placement. The students choose the speciality in which they wish to work and arrange the placement themselves. Many choose to work abroad, or in areas of healthcare not previously encountered in their own clinical education.

■ Current issues

Technology in physiotherapy

Enter the words 'physiotherapy' and 'news' into an internet search engine and most of the links that you get are to news stories about new forms of treatment. Although the basic techniques used in physiotherapy have been around for a long time – physical manipulation, repetition of exercises and other forms of manual therapy – technology plays an increasing part.

Probably the most widely used application of technology within physiotherapy is ultrasound. Ultrasound treatment utilises high-frequency (up to 3MHz – too high for the human ear to hear) sound waves. Ultrasound is used extensively in medicine for diagnosis, either to form images in order to see what is happening inside the body (for instance, scans that show a foetus inside the womb) or to measure blood flow. Whenever ultrasound waves pass from one tissue to another a small percentage of the beam is reflected back, and these reflected sound waves are used to create a picture, or to measure the speed at which blood is flowing (using something called the Doppler Effect).

Ultrasound can also be used therapeutically, that is, for treatment. It has been used to accelerate tissue repair and to relieve pain since the 1950s. It is used to treat a variety of conditions such as sports injuries, sprains, tendonitis, arthritis and ulcers, and to relieve the pain associated with, for instance, phantom limbs in amputees. The sound waves penetrate deep into the body and, although the biological effects are not completely understood, it is likely that the vibration caused by the sound waves produces a combination of heating (thermal effects) and stimulation of tissue and blood vessels (mechanical effects). Ultrasound is usually given at the end of a course of treatment, following other forms of manual therapy.

Ultrasound equipment is relatively cheap to buy (less than £2000 for an ultrasound machine) and is easy to use. The total cost to the NHS of ultrasound in physiotherapy is around £5 million per year – a tiny proportion of the total NHS bill. The drawbacks of the extensive use of ultrasound in physiotherapy are that there is little conclusive clinical evidence that it is effective; and that there is a possible risk of tissue damage if the power settings on individual machines are not accurately calibrated.

Another treatment that utilises sound waves, extracorporeal shockwave therapy (ESWT), is being introduced into physiotherapy clinics. ESWT was brought to a wider audience in 2004 when Sachin Tendulkar, the Indian cricketer, received shockwave therapy to treat tennis elbow which had failed to respond to conventional physiotherapy. Developed from the devices that generate pulses of sound waves to destroy kidney stones, ESWT devices produce pulses of high-pressure sound that travel through the skin. Soft tissue and bone that are subjected to these pulses of high-pressure energy heal back stronger. Tennis elbow results from calcification of a tendon and is usually treated with mechanical exercise or steroid injection (which risk weakening the tendon still further), but new treatments are also being developed (see page 59).

Increasingly, robots are being used in physiotherapy. This does not mean that next time you require physiotherapy you will be treated by R2-D2, Bender or Kryton. The effective rehabilitation of patients with cerebral palsy, or following a stroke or other brain injuries, requires repetitive movement exercises and controllable resistance to motion. In one such treatment the patient is coupled to a robot joystick that guides him or her through a series of movements. The robot can be programmed to vary the scope of the movement, to increase or decrease the resistance, or to help the patient to complete the movements. To increase interest levels for the patient the movements can be integrated into a 'game' on a screen in front of the patient. In this way tens of thousands of therapeutic movements can be completed over the course of a few weeks – far more than the physiotherapist could manage, and more than the patient is likely to be able to accomplish alone. Virtual reality is also used to alleviate the boredom often associated with repetitive exercises. Patients can 'put' themselves into a virtual reality environment where they can take part in a game that requires them to perform the necessary therapeutic movements.

RSI

Repetitive Strain Injury, or RSI, is an increasingly common complaint amongst computer users. As the name suggests, the condition is caused by repetition of certain movements, usually associated with computer keyboard use. However, it is not confined to computer users, and has been diagnosed in many people whose jobs involve manual labour or machine operation. The condition can also occur when the person's posture is inappropriate to the task that he or she is undertaking. RSI manifests itself as pain, mostly when the task that caused it is being carried out, but often at other times as well. It usually affects the neck, shoulders, elbows, wrists or hands. RSI is also known by other names including Repetitive Stress Injury, WMSD (work-related musculoskeletal disorder), WRULD (work-related upper limb disorder), CTD (cumulative trauma disorder) and OOS (occupational overuse syndrome).

The term RSI actually encompasses a number of different conditions, most commonly Carpal Tunnel Syndrome. *Carpus* comes from the Greek word *karpos*, which means wrist. The joint in the wrist is surrounded by fibrous tissue, and there is a small gap between this tissue and the bone, through which a nerve (the median nerve) passes. The nerve then splits to serve the fingers and thumb. Repetitive movement of the wrist can cause swelling of the tissue in the wrist, putting pressure on the median nerve. Symptoms include numbness and tingling in the fingers and thumb, followed by pain. The condition can usually be cured by a combination of physiotherapy and rest.

People who work in factories are three times more likely to get RSI than office workers, reports the CSP. They say that 'Over 370,000 people in Great Britain are afflicted with Repetitive Strain Injury and as many as 86,000 new cases were recorded last year. In terms of employee absence, lower productivity and staff turnover, the cost to employers is nearly £300 million!'

The CSP website reports that the Labour Research Department analysed Health and Safety Executive figures for the CSP and discovered that metal, plastics, textile and other plant and machine workers (1.1 per 100 workers) were the most likely to get RSI, followed by bricklayers, plumbers, carpenters and others in skilled trades (0.91 per 100 workers). Professionals (0.32) and managers (0.36) were least likely to get RSI.

Not everyone believes that RSI actually exists. Carpal Tunnel Syndrome certainly does and can be caused by obesity, arthritis, diabetes and pregnancy, but there are those who are sceptical as to whether repetitive movement is a cause. A report in the *British Medical Journal* on research done at Manchester University cast some doubts about RSI. The research indicated that the majority of those who suffered from arm or wrist pain (105 people in a survey encompassing 1200 volunteers) were also the most dissatisfied with their jobs and suffered from high stress levels. In other words, the pain could be due to psychological or stress factors rather than simply the physical aspects of their jobs.

Rehabilitation of stroke patients

A stroke occurs when a blood clot blocks a blood vessel in the brain, causing brain cells in the area to die. If treatment is not given immediately, further cells in the surrounding areas also die. The functions, such as speech, memory or movement that were controlled by these brain cells are then affected, depending on the area of the brain where the blood vessels were blocked. The severity of the stroke can vary from patient to patient, and the effects may be very minor (and temporary) or they may lead to paralysis or death.

The main types of rehabilitation are:

- Physical therapy – to improve mechanical skills such as walking, use of the hands, or balance.
- Occupational therapy – to re-learn the skills that are required for everyday life such as eating, dressing and looking after oneself.
- Speech therapy – to re-learn how to communicate effectively.

Physiotherapy for stroke patients must begin as early as possible following the stroke in order to be effective. Improvement is slow and recovery is difficult six months after the stroke. However, paralysed muscles must not be treated too early or they may be permanently damaged. Research carried out at the University of Texas, reported in *New Scientist*, found that rats and monkeys which had received small brain injuries to cause paralysis of a limb suffered further injury if treatment was started immediately. The researchers surmised that glutamate, a neurotransmitter that is released during movement, was the probable cause since, in large concentrations, it acts as a toxin. Brain damage appeared to multiply its effects. Research is now being carried out to find drugs that will block the effects of glutamate.

The expertise of the physiotherapist is vital in assessing when (and in what form) treatment should start. At the start of the treatment, the physiotherapist will prepare muscles for the more intensive treatments that will follow, and will work on enabling the patient to support his or her own weight if leg muscles are affected. The later stages of physiotherapy may involve compensation for permanently damaged muscles through the introduction of aids such as walking frames. The physiotherapist may work alongside occupational therapists, speech therapists, carers and psychologists to try to prepare the patient for a return to 'normal' life.

Exercise referral schemes

Introduced 10 years ago, NHS exercise referral schemes have become increasingly popular. In 2004 the government outlined proposals to provide GPs with national standards for 'prescribing' exercise programmes for their patients.

Exercise referral schemes are used to help patients suffering from a wide range of problems, including:

■ Coronary heart disease
■ Hypertension
■ Obesity
■ Diabetes
■ Mental health problems, including depression
■ Musculo-skeletal problems, eg chronic low-back pain
■ Problems caused by falls.

In July 2004, the CSP published figures showing that the number of schemes has mushroomed by over 500% during the last decade. In 1994, there were 157 exercise referral schemes in existence, compared to the latest estimate of 816. The Chief Executive of the CSP, quoted on the CSP website, said 'This report highlights the way in which exercise referral schemes are of particular benefit to patients at risk of heart attack and stroke. They are also helping people successfully tackle obesity, diabetes, mental health problems and low-back pain. Physiotherapists play crucial roles in the prevention and management of these conditions and are ideally placed to help roll out a wider network of schemes.'

Andree Dean, Executive Chair of the Fitness Industry Association, welcomed the initiative:'Exercise referral schemes provide great opportunities for fitness professionals to work in partnership with health professionals on schemes that target people who do not normally take exercise. These can make a real contribution to public health.'

Alternative therapies

Physiotherapists are now becoming increasingly interested in utilising so-called 'alternative therapies' alongside traditional techniques. These can include:

■ Acupuncture
■ Alexander technique
■ Aromatherapy
■ Chiropractic medicine
■ Reflex therapy
■ Massage.

Acupuncture

Acupuncture originated over 3000 years ago in China. The practitioner inserts thin needles into the body at designated places in order to help to alleviate or cure problems. Nowadays, this may also involve small electric currents. It is thought that the needles stimulate the body's nervous system into producing its own painkilling substances.

The safe delivery of acupuncture is monitored by the the Acupuncture Association of Chartered Physiotherapists (AACP), a clinical interest group of the Chartered Society of Physiotherapy.

Massage

Massage is the manipulation of the soft parts of the body.

Physiotherapists with a particular interest can do postgraduate training in many different types of massage. The CSP has a special interest group: Chartered Physiotherapists Interested in Massage & Soft Tissue Therapies (CPMaSTT).

Reflex therapy

Reflex therapy deals with problems within the body by targeting related points on, for example, the feet, hands or head. Reflex therapy can be arranged by consulting a chartered physiotherapist who is a member of the Association of Chartered Physiotherapists in Reflex Therapy (ACPIRT), the clinical interest group of the Chartered Society of Physiotherapy.

Alexander technique

The Alexander technique is a method of releasing unwanted muscular tension throughout the body by making the patient aware of balance, posture and co-ordination while performing everyday actions.

Aromatherapy

Aromatherapy uses essential oils that are derived from plants and flowers. The oils are either vapourised and inhaled, or applied directly to the body – often in conjunction with massage.

Chiropractic medicine

Chiropractic medicine aims to address the improper alignment of the vertebrae in the spinal which, it is believed, causes a number of physical disorders. This is achieved by manipulation.

◼ Employment prospects

Whilst the experience of many patients who are referred to hospitals for physiotherapy treatment and who face long waiting lists would suggest that there is a shortage of NHS physiotherapists, a recent survey by the CSP revealed that of the 2000 or so physiotherapy graduates who left university in 2005, about 53% did not have jobs to go to after graduation. The Hospital Episode Statistics for 2003/04 reveal the need for more NHS physiotherapists, says the CSP: 'Over half a million people with injuries were admitted to an NHS hospital in England last year. They waited anywhere between 26 days to be admitted for injuries to the elbow and forearm, to a massive 76 days for knee and lower leg injuries.' The picture is not quite as bleak as it seems, however, as most physiotherapy graduates find relevant employment eventually and, once you have a job, promotion prospects are good, with many vacancies at senior level.

■ Continuing Professional Development (CPD)

Throughout their careers physiotherapists are expected to develop their skills and to keep up to date with developments within the field in a structured and systematic way. This is known as CPD. Physiotherapists are responsible for identifying, planning and recording their own CPD, setting themselves targets and collecting evidence in a portfolio to support their CPD.

The process of CPD is summarised in the diagram below:

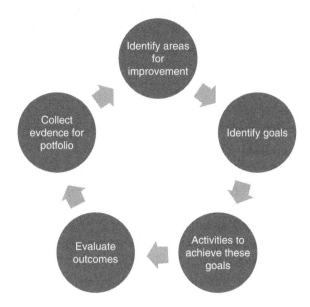

Related courses

Occupational therapy

Occupational therapists help people to carry out the tasks and activities that are necessary for them to lead a fulfilling life. These might be work related – helping people with disabilities to cope with their jobs; or these might be everyday things like cooking, bathing, travelling or socialising. Occupational therapists work in hospitals, for charities and social organisations, in schools and the workplace, in prisons, within the local community, and in many other situations. Occupational therapists deal with physical, mental and social needs, for example:

■ Helping children deal with learning difficulties
■ Helping people with mental illness to look after themselves, or to be successful in their jobs

- Working with accident victims to enable them to re-learn physical tasks
- Advising businesses about how to adapt facilities and premises to enable people with disabilities to cope with their jobs
- Creating rehabilitation programmes for refugees or the homeless.

To practise as an occupational therapist, it is necessary to follow a degree course in Occupational Therapy (COT), which has been approved by the HPC, and accredited by the College of Occupational Therapists. For UK students, the tuition fees for the degree course are normally paid by the NHS. Contact details for the COT and other useful organisations can found in on pages 55–7.

Courses and grade requirements

You are advised to check the *UCAS Handbook* or website for information on courses and universities before applying.

University of Birmingham
Tel: 0121 415 8900
Website: www.bham.ac.uk

Bournemouth University
Tel: 01202 524111
Website: www.bournemouth.ac.uk

University of Bradford
Tel: 01274 233081
Website: www.brad.ac.uk

University of Brighton
Tel: 01273 600900
Website: www.brighton.ac.uk

Bristol, University of the West of England
Tel: 0117 344333
Website: www.uwe.ac.uk

Brunel University
Tel: 01895 265265
Website: www.brunel.ac.uk

Cardiff University
Tel: 029 2087 9999
Website: www.cardiff.ac.uk

University of Central Lancashire
Tel: 01772 201201
Website: www.uclan.ac.uk

Coventry University
Tel: 024 7688 7688
Website: www.coventry.ac.uk

University of East Anglia
Tel: 01603 456161
Website: www.uea.ac.uk

University of East London
Tel: 020 8223 2835
Website: www.uel.ac.uk

Glasgow Caledonian University
Tel: 0141 331 3000
Website: www.gcal.ac.uk

University of Hertfordshire
Tel: 01707 284800
Website: www.herts.ac.uk

University of Huddersfield
Tel: 01484 422288
Website: www.hud.ac.uk

Keele University
Tel: 01782 584005
Website: www.keele.ac.uk

King's College, University of London
Tel: 020 7836 5454
Website: www.kcl.ac.uk

Leeds Metropolitan University
Tel: 0113 283 3113
Website: www.leedsmet.ac.uk

University of Liverpool
Tel: 0151 794 2000
Website: www.liv.ac.uk

Manchester Metropolitan University
Tel: 0161 247 2459
Website: www.mmu.ac.uk

Northumbria University
Tel: 0191 232 6002
Website: www.northumbria.ac.uk

University of Nottingham
Tel: 0115 951 5151
Website: www.nottingham.ac.uk

Oxford Brookes University
Tel: 01865 483040
Website: www.brookes.ac.uk

University of Plymouth
Tel: 01752 232137
Website: www.plymouth.ac.uk

Queen Margaret University College, Edinburgh
Tel: 0131 317 3247
Website: www.qmuc.ac.uk

Robert Gordon University, Aberdeen
Tel: 01224 262728
Website: www.rgu.ac.uk

University of Salford
Tel: 0161 295 4545
Website: www.salford.ac.uk

Sheffield Hallam University
Tel: 0114 225 5555
Website: www.shu.ac.uk

University of Southampton
Tel: 023 8059 5000
Website: www.soton.ac.uk

St George's Hospital Medical School
Tel: 020 8725 5201
Website: www.sghms.ac.uk

University of Teesside
Tel: 01642 218121
Website: www.tees.ac.uk

University of Ulster
Tel: 028 7032 4221
Website: www.ulster.ac.uk

York St John College
Tel: 01904 624624
Website: www.yorksj.ac.uk

Grade and subject requirements for 2008

The grade requirements listed here are correct at the time of going to press. Contact the universities before completing your application to check that they are unchanged.

Institution	A2 Tariff/Grades*	A2 Biology?**
Birmingham	ABB	Grade B
Bournemouth	300	Preferred
Bradford	BBB	Grade B

Brighton	BBB	Grade B
Bristol UWE	280–340	Yes
Brunel	280	Grade B
Cardiff	AAB	Grade B
Central Lancashire	BBB	1 science
Coventry	BBB	Grade B
East Anglia	300	Grade B
East London	300	1 science
Glasgow Caledonian	BBB	1 science/Maths
Hertfordshire	300	2 life sciences
Huddersfield	BCC	Yes, or Sports Science/PE
Keele	ABB	Yes
King's College	BBBc	Yes, or 2 from Chemistry/Maths/Physics/Psychology
Leeds Met	280	1 science/Maths at B
Liverpool	BBB	Grade B
Manchester Met	BBB	1 biological science
Northumbria	320	Biological or behavioural science
Nottingham	ABB	Grade B, or PE grade B
Oxford Brookes	BBB	Grade B
Plymouth	300	Yes
Queen Margaret	ABB	2 from Biology/Maths/Chemistry/Physics
Robert Gordon	300	2 sciences
Salford	300	Grade B
Sheffield Hallam	300	Grade B in Biology or Chemistry
Southampton	ABBb	1 science
St George's	300	Grade B + another science
Teesside	300–320	Grade B
Ulster	BBB	1 science
York St John	300	Grade B

*   *Lower-case letters indicate additional grades required at AS level.*

** *Most universities will accept or even prefer Human Biology, and some will accept a biology-related subject (Psychology, Sports Science or PE), in place of Biology at A level. You should contact the university for details.*

■ Further reading/useful addresses

An essential starting point is the **Chartered Society of Physiotherapy's** website (www.csp.org.uk). It carries detailed information about careers in physiotherapy and recognised courses. The CSP also produces many useful booklets about physiotherapy. They can be contacted at: Chartered Society of Physiotherapy, 14 Bedford Row, London WC1R 4ED. Tel: 020 7306 6666; fax: 020 7306 6611. The CSP publishes a magazine, *Frontline*, aimed at practising physiotherapists. The magazine contains articles of interest and is a useful way of keeping up to date with current issues and new developments. There is also a large jobs section – a good way to make contact with physiotherapy practices if you are looking for work experience.

The **Irish Society of Chartered Physiotherapists**' website address is www.iscp.ie.

The **College of Occupational Therapists**, 106–114 Borough High Street, London SE1 1LB. Tel: 020 7357 6480; website: www.cot.co.uk.

The **Society of Chiropodists and Podiatrists**, 1 Fellmonger's Path, Tower Bridge Road, London SE1 3LY. Tel: 020 7234 8620; website: www.feetforlife.org.

For information on university applications contact UCAS (www.ucas. ac.uk). The UCAS website has a search facility that will enable you to check the latest entrance requirements for all universities that offer physiotherapy courses. Application materials can be obtained from UCAS, PO Box 28, Cheltenham, Gloucestershire GL50 3SA.

For detailed information on all physiotherapy courses consult *Degree Course Offers* written by Brian Heap and published by Trotman (Tel: 020 8484 1150; website: www.trotman.co.uk).

Other useful addresses

NHS (England) Student Grants Unit
NHS Pensions Agency
200-220 Broadway
Fleetwood
Lancashire FY7 8SS
Tel: 0845 358 6655
Fax: 0125 377 4491
E-mail: enquiries@nhspa.gov.uk
Website: www.nhsstudentgrants.co.uk

Department for Employment and Learning
Northern Ireland
Student Support Branch
4th Floor, Adelaide House
39-49 Adelaide Street
Belfast BT2 8FD
Tel: 028 9025 7777
Website: www.delni.gov.uk

Students Awards Agency for Scotland
3 Redheughs Rigg
South Gyle
Edinburgh EH12 9HH
Tel: 0131 4768212
Website: www.student-support-saas.gov.uk

NHS (Wales) Students Awards Unit
2nd Floor, Golate House
101 St Mary Street
Cardiff CF10 1DX
Tel: 029 2026 1495
Fax: 029 2026 1499
www.wales.nhs.uk

NHS (Cymru) Uned Dyfarniadau Myfyrwyr
2il Lawr, Ty Golate
101 Heol Eglwys Fair
Caerdydd
CF10 1DX
Ffôn: 029 2026 1495
Facs: 029 2026 1499

For visually-impaired applicants
RNIB Physiotherapy Resource Centre
University of East London
Romford Road
London E15 4LZ
Telephone: 020 8223 4950
Fax: 020 8223 4954
www.uel.ac.uk/rnib/is

Jane S Owen Hutchinson, Manager
RNIB Physiotherapy Support Service
Mobile: 07748 657457
E-mail: jane.owenhutchinson@rnib.org.uk
E-mail: k.a.atkinson@uel.ac.uk

Examination boards
www.ocr.org.uk
www.edexcel.org.uk
www.aqa.org.uk
www.wjec.co.uk

Online physiotherapy information
www.library.nhs.uk/
www.emedicine.com/pmr/contents.htm
www.onthegophysio.com
www.therapyweekly.co.uk

www.thephysiotherapysite.co.uk
www.metis-uk.com

University league tables
www.timesonline.co.uk
http://education.guardian.co.uk/universityguide

Books on careers/university applications
Degree Course Offers, **Brian Heap, Trotman**
Getting into Physiotherapy, **Trotman**
How to Complete Your UCAS Application, **MPW Guides/Trotman**
The Mature Students' Directory 2004, **Trotman**
University and College Entrance: The Official Guide, **UCAS**

Books on physiotherapy
There are numerous textbooks covering all aspects of physiotherapy. Most of these are aimed at undergraduates or physiotherapy professionals. The following will give A level (or the equivalent) students an overview of what studying physiotherapy would entail:

Principles and Practice of Physical Therapy, William Arnold-Taylor, Stanley Thornes

A Practical Guide to Sports Injuries, Malcolm T F Read, Butterworth Heinemann

■ Postscript

If you have any comments or questions arising out of this book, we and the staff of MPW would be very happy to answer them. You can contact us at the addresses below.

Good luck with your applications!

James Burnett
MPW (London)
90-92 Queen's Gate
London SW7 5AB
Tel: 020 7835 1355
Fax: 020 7259 2705
E-mail: enquiries@mpw.co.uk

MPW (Cambridge)
3-4 Brookside
Cambridge CB2 1JE
Tel: 01223 350158
Fax: 01223 366429
E-mail: enquiries@cambridge.mpw.co.uk

MPW (Birmingham)
38 Highfield Road
Edgbaston
Birmingham B15 3ED
Tel: 0121 454 9637
Fax: 0121 454 6433
E-mail: enq@birmingham.mpw.co.uk